Hiking and Hydration
Natural Nutrition that Boosts your Stamina

Table of Contents

Chapter 1. Introduction

Embark on an invigorating journey of discovery with our special report: "Hiking and Hydration: Natural Nutrition that Boosts your Stamina". Uncover the secrets of staying energized and focused when tackling those challenging trails, all while enjoying the serenity of Mother Nature. This user-friendly guide, filled with vibrant insights, takes you through the importance of maintaining hydration and harnessing the power of natural nutrition to supercharge your endurance. The call of the wild is beckoning, and we're here to equip you with the knowledge you need, not just to answer it, but to do so with gusto and vitality. Devour the contents of this engaging report and, as you lace up your hiking boots, you'll also be packing a reservoir of newfound wisdom and confidence.

Chapter 2. Introduction to Hiking and Hydration

Welcome to the realm of wellness that lies off the beaten path. Even when it feels as though our existence consists of endless concrete plains and interminable rat races, a verdant wilderness nestled amidst secluded serenity waits patiently to be discovered. An ecosystem, charging your vitality as a hiker, rings with the whispers of birdsongs, the rustle of leaves underfoot, and the tranquil flow of a nearby stream. But to experience its magnificence, the body, mind, and spirit must resonate on a wavelength that matches the exuberance of nature's bounty.

2.1. Hiking: A Journey Into the Wilderness

In the visceral allure of nature, there lie rugged trails that bring out their beauty, encapsulating the perennial symphony of the life force pulsating in the great outdoors. To embark upon these pathways is a pleasure you owe to yourself; to discover stretch goals, appreciation for the subtle rhythms of nature, and treasures bundled in the heart of the wilderness.

As you lace up your boots, fixate your backpack, and set off for a rendezvous with the unknown, you expose yourself to the realm of enthusiasm, passion, and the unsaid, waiting to spring upon you. The trails, unbeknownst to many, are your teachers. They enhance your perseverance, enrich your spirit, and fill your senses with unparalleled joy and serenity.

2.2. A Trekker's Relationship with Hydration

Mundane as it may seem, hydration forms the cornerstone of any successful hiking or trekking expedition. In spite of this, many hikers overlook its importance and often find themselves constrained in the wilderness, the lack of water wreaking havoc on their carefully planned schedules.

As your ally, water serves an array of purposes. Not only does it quench your thirst and replenish lost fluids, it also cools your body, aids digestion, cushions your joints, and helps your body flush out wastes. Lack of proper hydration can lead to acute difficulties such as fatigue, headache, confusion, and, at worst, heatstroke. Thus, to ignore the call for hydration is at your peril.

2.3. Answering the Call for Hydration

In order to respond to the body's SOS, it's essential to understand the physiological signals of dehydration. With symptoms ranging from increased thirst and dry mouth to fatigue and lightheadedness, it's an imbalance that slowly creeps into your system. Dehydration can impair your attention, reduce your coordination, and decrease your physical performance. Consequences such as muscle cramps, nausea, and rapid heartbeat can interfere with the joy of your hiking experience.

Preparing your body for the hike isn't simply about filling your flask at the start of the hike. It's about maintaining a regimen of regular fluid intake before, during, and after the hike. Hydration should be gradual and consistent, as gulping down water causes the body to dispose of the surplus by increasing urine production, thereby losing valuable minerals.

2.4. Natural Nutrition as Nature's Elixir

In addition to staying hydrated, it's essential to feed the body with the fuel it needs. Dietary choices play a significant role in keeping you energized and in peak form. A balance of carbohydrates, proteins, and fats should be the central idea of the hiker's meal plan.

Fruits, nuts, seeds, vegetables, and contemporary superfoods offer a power-packed blend of essential nutrients that serve as fuel for your body. These foods are lightweight, non-perishable, and rich in energy, making them perfect for your hiking backpack.

The culmination of this distinct world of hydration and natural nutrition leads to a successful and enjoyable hiking journey. The communion with nature enhances the joy of the trail, but only when you come prepared and equipped. Ensure you bring with you an understanding of the unspoken pact of hydration and nutrition to truly appreciate the invigorating adventures that Mother Nature has in store for you.

Chapter 3. Fundamentals of Hydration Science

When we embark on a hiking journey, staying adequately hydrated is equally as important as lacing up the proper footwear. Behind this fundamental principle lies a body of fascinating science. The study of hydration science reveals not only why we need to keep our bodies hydrated but also how best to accomplish this, particularly when planning for physically demanding excursions such as hiking.

3.1. The Basics of Hydration

Water, our primary hydration source, plays a critical role in maintaining the body's metabolic and physiological functions. It helps regulate body temperature, facilitates digestion, supports nutrient absorption and transportation, and even aids cognitive functions. However, the body continually loses water through sweating, breathing, and excreting wastes, making regular replenishment crucial.

Expectedly, when you engage in strenuous activities such as hiking, your body's demand for water escalates significantly. Sweating, a natural cooling mechanism, intensifies, leading to greater water and essential electrolyte losses. This emphasizes the necessity of staying ahead of your body's hydration needs during these activities.

3.2. Understanding Dehydration

Dehydration occurs when water output exceeds intake. In a dehydrated state, the body struggles to perform its normal functions, which can cause a slew of symptoms. This range from mild symptoms like increased thirst, dry mouth, fatigue, and decreased urine output, to acute problems like dizziness, confusion, rapid heartbeat or breathing. Sustained dehydration could lead to severe health problems such as heat injuries, kidney issues, and shock.

Understanding how the body signals dehydration is important. Thirst, although a common indicator, may not be a reliable signal during intensive physical activities. Sometimes, when you finally feel thirsty, you're already significantly dehydrated. Recognizing non-thirst symptoms early can help prompt timely hydration and prevent serious complications.

3.3. Hydration Requirements

Everyone's hydration needs are unique and are influenced by factors like age, sex, weight, and activity levels. Climatic conditions, altitude, and the nature of the hike (intensity and duration) also have a role in determining a hiker's hydration demand. However, a general rule of thumb suggests consuming around 0.5 to 1 liter of water for every hour of hiking.

Note, the body's capacity to absorb water is limited. Consuming large quantities in short periods can lead to hyponatremia, a condition where the body's sodium levels are dangerously low. This underscores the importance of sipping small quantities of water throughout your hike.

3.4. Role of Electrolytes

Hydration is not just about water. When the body excretes sweat, it is also losing essential compounds known as electrolytes. Sodium, potassium, calcium, and magnesium are key electrolytes that play vital roles in muscle function, nerve signalling, and maintaining the body's pH balance.

Replacing lost electrolytes is as crucial as replenishing water. Consuming electrolyte-infused waters or sports drinks, or snacking on electrolyte-rich foods while hiking can help your body maintain the necessary electrolyte balance.

3.5. Strategies for Hydration

Now that the importance of hydration and the associated risks of dehydration are clear, how can hikers ensure they stay appropriately hydrated?

1. Devise a Hydration Plan: Having a hydration strategy before you start the hike is useful. This should account for the trail's length and difficulty, the climate, and personal factors such as your sweat rate.

2. Hydrate Before Hiking: Start the hydration process even before the hike begins. Drink plenty of water and electrolyte-rich foods or drinks prior to setting out.

3. Regular Fluid Intake: As you hike, consume small amounts of water frequently to avoid dehydration.

4. Consider Your Meals: Plan your meals to incorporate moisture-rich foods that can contribute to your hydration efforts.

5. Stay Alert to Body Signals: Pay attention to signs of dehydration and adjust your water intake as needed.

The art and science of staying hydrated while hiking is a vital part of the adventure. As we delve deeper into this, remember that fine-tuning your hydration habits for optimal stamina and performance is a process of continual learning and adjustment.

The road to mastering hydration might seem overwhelming, but consider it an essential part of your hiking gear. As you keep taking strides, you'll find not just the right balance, but also an enhanced hiking experience full of vigor and enjoyment. Hydrated bodies make happy hikers!

Chapter 4. Connecting Hydration and Stamina

As we begin our exploration of maintaining hydration and stamina, it is important to lay the foundation by defining key terms, outlining how our bodies function, and exploring why hydration is crucial for endurance. We embark on this educational journey with the same mindset we would apply to hiking – one step at a time, curious, and open to absorbing knowledge along the way.

4.1. Understanding Hydration and Stamina

Hydration refers to the process by which water is added to keep something moist. In this context, it is about how our bodies absorb, distribute, and maintain fluids. On the other side, stamina is the body's ability to endure an effort for a particular period of time. Stamina is inherently linked to endurance, as it defines the body's power to withstand fatigue or resist disease. On the surface, these two concepts might seem distinct, but upon further exploration, we discover their intertwined relationship.

4.2. The Anatomy of Hydration

Water is not just a thirst quencher; it is a vital building block of life, responsible for enabling almost all biological processes. When we talk about hydration, we are essentially referring to maintaining an optimal fluid balance in our body. This balance plays an important role in functions such as heat regulation, cushioning organs and joints, maintaining skin health, aiding digestion, and removing waste.

4.3. Why Hydration Matters for Stamina

We have established that water is much more than just a refreshing beverage. Its benefits extend to supporting physical stamina. During physical exertion, our bodies produce heat, which results in sweat to cool us down. This is an efficient system, but one that draws heavily on our water stores. Therefore, by staying hydrated, we replace lost fluids, maintain an optimum body temperature, and prevent the adverse effects of dehydration, such as muscle fatigue, light-headedness, and reduced coordination – all of which are enemies of stamina.

4.4. Dehydration: Consequences and Symptoms

Understanding dehydration is crucial to comprehend the relationship between hydration and stamina. Dehydration occurs when the amount of water leaving the body is greater than the amount being consumed. Symptoms can range from mild, such as thirst and dry mouth, to severe, like muscle cramps, rapid heart rate, and extreme fatigue. On a performance spectrum, dehydration not only decreases physical ability but also impairs cognitive function, reducing both physical and mental stamina.

4.5. Hydration Techniques for Enhancing Stamina

Now that we know hydration's integral role in maintaining stamina, the question that arises is - how do we stay hydrated? Here are some insights:

1. Pre-Hydrate: Drink fluids such as water or sports drinks before

exertion to ensure your body starts off in an optimal state.

2. Sip Constantly: Avoid guzzling large amounts at once. Instead, drink small amounts frequently to maintain regular hydration levels.

3. Listen to Your Body: Thirst is a late response to dehydration. So, make sure to keep drinking even if you don't feel the immediate need.

4. Eat Your Hydration: Certain foods, especially fruits and vegetables like watermelon and cucumber, offer significant fluid content along with vitamins, minerals, and electrolytes.

5. Post-Hydrate: Replenishing fluids after physical endeavors is crucial to recovery and readiness for the next round of exertion.

4.6. The Power of Electrolytes

While drinking water is key, it's not the only method to preserve our stamina. Electrolytes, minerals found in our bodily fluids, can make a big difference. Electrolytes maintain fluid balance and replace critical nutrients such as sodium, potassium, and magnesium, lost through sweat. They not only help maintain hydration but also regulate nerve and muscle function and pH levels. Here's where sports drinks or specially purposed water can come into play. Note that most electrolyte drinks are high in sugar and should be chosen with caution.

4.7. Natural Nutrition to Complement Hydration

What we consume also plays a central role in maintaining hydration and amplifying stamina. Foods rich in proteins, wholesome carbohydrates, and healthy fats provide long-lasting energy and can enhance endurance. Among these, whole grains, lean meats (like chicken and fish), nuts, and fruits like bananas are particularly beneficial due to their nutrient-packed composition.

4.8. Hydration for Extended Hikes

Long hikes present special challenges. It isn't feasible to carry enormous amounts of water, and streams or rivers may not always be nearby. Here, equipment like hydration bladders or portable water purifiers comes in handy. Also, prepare by studying the area ahead of time and knowing where natural water sources are located.

This comprehensive understanding of hydration and its correlation with stamina equips you to approach your mountain trails or extended hikes with the required know-how. Remember, your body is the best judge, so pay close attention to its signals. Here's to your hydrated and enduring adventures. After all, that peak isn't going to climb itself!

Chapter 5. Top Hydrating Foods for Hikers

Hydration is not only about gulping down several liters of water a day - it's also about consuming the right foods. Certain foods, due to their high water content and nutritional value, can assist in maintaining a robust hydration balance while providing necessary energy on the trails. Next, we'll explore some of the top hydrating foods that should form an integral part of any hiker's food pack.

5.1. Water-Rich Fruits and Vegetables

Fruits and vegetables contain mostly water, making them ideal for a hydration-focused diet. They're lightweight, making them perfect companions on a hiking trail. Furthermore, they provide crucial vitamins and minerals, fiber, and antioxidants to keep you healthy and energetic.

1. Cucumbers: Comprising 96% water, cucumbers hold the top rank when it comes to hydrating foods. Also rich in vitamin K, cucumbers aid in bone health.

2. Watermelon: Aptly named, these juicy treats are 92% water and also provide a healthy dose of vitamins A and C, as well as inflammation-fighting antioxidants.

3. Strawberries: These tasty fruits are 91% water. They're loaded with vitamins, minerals, and antioxidants.

4. Celery: With a water content of about 95%, celery is an excellent hydrating food. It also provides a good amount of fiber and Vitamin K.

5. Oranges: Known for their rich vitamin C content, oranges are also

88% water, providing hydration along with the energy from natural sugars.

5.2. Energy-Packed Nuts and Seeds

Though not typically known for their water content, certain nuts and seeds are prized among outdoor adventurers for their nutrient-rich, long-lasting, energy-providing abilities. They also facilitate hydration by helping to maintain electrolyte balance.

1. Almonds: Packed with healthy fats, protein, and fiber, almonds are perfect for a quick energy boost. They also contain good amounts of vitamin E and magnesium.

2. Walnuts: They offer a plant-based source of omega-3 fatty acids along with other useful nutrients beneficial for brain health and inflammation reduction.

3. Chia Seeds: When soaked, chia seeds can absorb up to 12 times their weight in water, becoming a gel that helps prolong hydration and retain electrolytes.

4. Pumpkin Seeds: High in magnesium, these seeds help with energy production and are great for heart health.

5.3. Rehydration Through Meals

While it's essential to snack on hydrating foods throughout the day, it's equally important to enjoy heartily hydrating meals. Here are some trail-friendly meal ideas:

1. Quinoa Salad: Made ahead of time, a cold quinoa salad with a variety of vegetables provides plenty of hydration and fiber. Moreover, quinoa is a complete protein source.

2. Rice and Beans: This classic combo provides complex carbs for long-term energy and fiber to support digestion. Use precooked

and dehydrated ingredients to ensure light packing.

3. Pasta Primavera: It's an excellent dinner option on the trail. With pasta, you have an excellent carb source, while the vegetables provide hydration, fiber, vitamins, and minerals.

5.4. Portable Hydration Boosters

Apart from food, there are a few other innovative ways to maintain your hydration.

1. Hydration mix tablets: These are light, portable, and packed with electrolytes. Simply add it to your water bottle to create a hydrating, tasteful drink.

2. Green tea bags: Rich in antioxidants, green tea can help combat inflammation and provide gentle, sustained energy. The hot brew also aids in maintaining body heat in colder environments.

3. Rehydration salts: Available in packets, these salts are a mix of glucose and electrolytes. It's a quick fix to recover from intense dehydration.

It's crucial to note that hydration strategy should be personalized based on the intensity and duration of the hike, weather conditions, and individual metabolic considerations. Remember, staying hydrated is not merely about quenching your thirst but ensuring your body has the required nourishment and resources it needs to perform optimally throughout your hiking journey. Drink water, eat healthily, and allow the natural strength from good hydration habits guide you through the trails.

Chapter 6. Natural Drinks That Fuel Endurance

A successful hike isn't just about lacing up your boots and hitting the trail. It's equally important to ensure your body is properly fueled and hydrated to endure the physical challenge that lies ahead. Choosing natural drinks rich in the right nutrients can dramatically enhance your stamina and endurance.

6.1. Understanding Hydration and Energy

Before diving into natural drinks for endurance, let's first grasp the intimate relationship between hydration and energy. Your body heavily relies on water for all its critical functions, including the delivery of nutrients to cells and the removal of waste products. With adequate hydration, your muscles function at their peak, leading to improved stamina and reduced fatigue. Water is also a fundamental component of blood, carrying the vital nutrients that provide energy to our cells.

During physical activity like hiking, your body loses fluids and essential minerals – electrolytes – through perspiration. This loss, if not adequately compensated, results in dehydration, causing decreased strength, endurance, and overall performance. Natural drinks come to the rescue, replenishing not only lost fluids but also necessary nutrients, ensuring a steady supply of energy and enhanced endurance.

6.2. The Power of Natural Drinks

While there's an abundance of energy drinks on the market, they often come loaded with artificial additives, sugars, and other undesirable ingredients. Natural drinks, on the other hand, provide hydration and energy in their purest form, benefiting your health beyond just boosting endurance.

Now, let's venture into the various natural drinks that are your best companions on hiking trails.

6.3. Water: The Ultimate Hydrator

It goes without saying that water is your number one ally in maintaining hydration. However, for extended physical activities like hiking, you might need more than just water to replace the electrolytes lost through sweat.

But that doesn't reduce the importance of regular water intake. Always begin your hiking day by drinking plenty of water. Likewise, carry an ample supply of it with you for the trail. A good rule of thumb is to drink half a liter of water every hour during the hike.

6.4. Coconut Water: Nature's Sports Drink

Coconut water is packed with electrolytes like potassium, magnesium, and sodium. This natural drink can be an excellent substitute for commercial sports drinks, providing hydration plus essential nutrients without the extra sugars and artificial ingredients often found in sports drinks. Coconut water also contains a good dose of vitamin C, which aids in strengthening immunity.

6.5. Herbal Teas: Loaded with Antioxidants

Herbal teas, especially those made from plants like green tea, hibiscus, and rooibos, are rich in antioxidants that can boost your overall health, improve heart health, and even enhance endurance and performance.

Green tea, in particular, includes a compound known as catechin, which can help you stay energized for longer. Try starting your day with a cup of green tea to energize your hike. Remember to let it cool down before packing, as hot liquids can lead to faster dehydration.

6.6. Fruit-infused Water: A Refreshing Twist

Adding a twist to your regular water by infusing it with fruits, spices, or herbs not only makes it flavorful but also adds a nutritional punch. Fruits like lemons, oranges, strawberries, or herbs like mint, can provide vitamins and antioxidants. For instance, lemon-infused water could deliver a quick vitamin C boost, which helps combat oxidative stress during a physically demanding activity like hiking.

6.7. Natural Juices: A Nutrient Powerhouse

Various fruits and vegetables can serve as a power-packed drink when juiced. Think citrus fruits like oranges and grapefruits, rich in vitamin C and electrolytes, or beetroot juice, which is known to enhance endurance and reduce fatigue.

Remember, while the whole fruit contains fiber that encourages slow absorption of sugars, juices deliver sugar more instantly. So, it's best to consume them in moderation to avoid energy crashes.

6.8. DIY Electrolyte Drinks: Tailor-Made for Your Convenience

You can make your batch of natural electrolyte drink at home, having control over the ingredients according to your taste and nutritional needs. A simple recipe could include water, freshly squeezed lemon or orange juice for vitamins and flavor, a pinch of Himalayan pink salt for electrolytes, and possibly a hint of natural sweetener like honey or maple syrup.

Maintaining a proper hydration strategy is critical for any outdoor activity. Furthermore, integrating natural beverages that are rich in essential nutrients into your hydration plan will significantly enhance your endurance. Experiment, mix and match, find what works best for you, and above all, enjoy the hike. The call of the wild is answered not just with strength and stamina, but with joy and an appreciation for the natural world surrounding us.

Chapter 7. Hydration Packs: Choosing the Best for You

Embarking into the wilderness, your mind filled with the call of the wild, the alluring beauty of nature waiting to be explored, can be truly exhilarating. Yet keeping your reservoir of endurance full is the key to making the most of this enthralling experience. And doing that, as we'll unravel in this chapter, is tightly linked with hydration and the pack you choose to carry your all-important water in.

7.1. Choosing the Perfect Hydration Pack

When it comes to choosing a hydration pack, there isn't a one-size-fits-all solution. Your ideal pack will depend upon your specific needs, the terrain you intend to explore, and the duration of your hike. Hence, the selection process must begin with understanding your requirements.

If you're planning for a strenuous day-long hike, the key features to look for are the pack's volume and water reservoir size. For shorter, more relaxed hikes, a smaller, lightweight backpack with a smaller reservoir could be more than sufficient. Importantly, comfort should never be compromised, regardless of the duration or terrain.

7.2. Paying Attention to the Size and Weight

The size and weight of the hydration pack you choose can greatly influence your hiking experience. Bulky packs could tire you out sooner, while lightweight packs, though more comfortable, may not be spacious enough to carry all your essentials.

Standard hydration packs come in three basic sizes: small (with a 1.5-liter water reservoir), medium (2-liter reservoir), and large (3-liter reservoir). If you're a casual hiker who enjoys short hikes, a small hydration pack should suffice. If you're an adventurous spirit who loves long hikes, opt for a larger hydration pack to ensure that you stay properly hydrated throughout.

7.3. Ergonomics and Hydration Pack Designs

Hydration packs generally come in two main designs - waist packs and backpacks. Waist packs are suitable for shorter, less strenuous hikes, while backpacks are a better fit for longer, more demanding walks in the wild. Choose a model that hugs your body comfortably and doesn't impede your freedom of movement.

Also consider the placement of the water tube on the pack. Some hikers prefer the tube on the right, while others find it more comfortable on the left. The best packs offer the option to shift the tube from one side to the other as per your preference.

7.4. Checking the Material Quality

The material quality of your hydration pack can impact both its lifespan and your comfort. High-quality materials make for durable packs that withstand wear and tear, while also providing better sweat management. Look for packs made from ripstop nylon or polyurethane for optimal durability and comfort.

Pay heed to the quality of the water bladder as well. It should be made from BPA-free, taste-free and odorless material to make your hydration experience enjoyable.

7.5. Evaluating the Cleaning Ease

Hydration packs need regular cleaning to keep the water fresh, and to prevent mold and bacteria growth. Cleaning ease largely depends on the design of the water reservoir and the tube. Wide-mouthed reservoirs that allow your hand to enter are the easiest to clean, and so are tubes that can be detached. Reservoirs and tubes that are dishwasher safe add to the cleaning ease.

7.6. Trying Before Buying

Remember to try on the hydration pack before buying it to check for fit and comfort. Put it on, adjust the straps and walk around a bit. It should feel snug and secure, without hampering your movement or causing discomfort.

So, as you pack your spirit of adventure and head out to answer the call of the wild, ensure you're well equipped with a well-chosen hydration pack. Sure, it's not the most glamorous bit of hiking gear, but it can be instrumental in making your hiking experience enjoyable, memorable, and safe. Choose it wisely, pack it rightly, and going the distance will be easy.

Chapter 8. Practical Tips for Staying Hydrated on the Trail

Proper hydration is not just about drinking water; rather, it's a thoughtful and organized mechanism your body requires, especially when embarking on physically demanding activities such as hiking.

8.1. The Importance of Hydration

When hiking, the body's demand for water increases. The body uses it to maintain its temperature, lubricate joints, and transport nutrients. When you're not adequately hydrated, your body's ability to perform these tasks decreases, deteriorating your physical performance and mental acuity. The symptoms of dehydration range from dizziness, fatigue, and headache to severe outcomes like heat stroke.

8.2. Quantifying Your Hydration Needs

Everyone's water needs differ. Factors such as your weight, physical condition, and the intensity and duration of the hike can influence how much water you should consume. A simple yet effective rule of thumb is to drink a half to one quart (approximately 0.5 to 1 liter) of water for every hour of hiking in moderate temperatures.

However, these quantities may increase in hotter climates or if you're on a strenuous hike. It's key to listen carefully to your body's signals of thirst and fatigue, and respond accordingly.

8.3. Hydration before Hiking

Hydration shouldn't start on the trail. It begins the day before you hike. Aim to drink about 4-6 glasses of water throughout the day before you embark on your hike, ensuring your body starts off well-hydrated.

In addition, your pre-hiking meal should include fruits and vegetables, which are naturally high in water content. Abstain from alcohol, as it can instigate dehydration. Wake up a bit earlier on your hiking day and drink 1-2 glasses of water about an hour before the hike starts.

8.4. Drinking Strategies During Hiking

Here's where many hikers get it wrong - drinking only when you are thirsty. If you wait until your throat is parched, your body is already hinting at dehydration. Regular and systematic drinking is pivotal.

Try to drink small amounts of water every 15-20 minutes, even if you're not feeling thirsty. This method keeps your body adequately hydrated without overloading your system. Also, always opt for cool, not cold water, as it absorbs faster.

8.5. Using Hydration Packs

Hydration packs offer convenience for hikers as they allow you to drink water while on the move, eliminating frequent stops. A pack with 2-3 liters capacity will keep you sufficiently hydrated for a moderate hike.

Remember to clean your hydration pack after every use, with a brush, warm water, and mild soap to prevent bacteria or mold buildup. Rinse it thoroughly and allow it to air dry before packing away.

8.6. Recognizing and Responding to Dehydration

Despite your best intentions, dehydration can creep in. Symptoms can include, but aren't limited to:

- Dry mouth and throat

- Fatigue and dizziness

- Dark, concentrated urine or less frequent urination

- Headache

- Rapid heartbeat and rapid breathing

If someone shows signs of dehydration, rehydrate them gradually with small sips of water. If symptoms persist, seek immediate medical attention.

8.7. Electrolyte Balance and Rehydration Salts

Water isn't enough to keep our bodies running optimally. When we sweat, we lose essential electrolytes such as sodium, potassium, and magnesium. Hydrating with water only can dilute these electrolytes in our body, leading to conditions like hyponatremia, also known as water intoxication.

Using rehydration salts or sports drinks can help replenish electrolytes lost during a strenuous hike. However, be cautious about drinks with high sugar content, as they can lead to an unnecessary calorie intake and possible dehydration.

8.8. Foods that Hydrate

Eating regular meals helps to restore the salts that you lose while sweating. Consume balanced hiking snacks like nuts, fresh or dried fruits, and cheese. These can help maintain your electrolyte balance. Moreover, certain foods, such as cucumber, watermelon, and oranges, have high water content, which can contribute to your hydration effort.

8.9. Importance of Rest

Rest plays an integral role in preventing dehydration. During breaks, seek out shade to prevent overheating, which can expedite dehydration. These intervals provide an excellent opportunity to drink your water, eat a nutritional snack, and assess how your body is handling the hiking trip.

Building these hydration strategies into your hiking habits will not only allow you to appreciate the trail's scenery better but also make it a more enjoyable and safe experience. Hydration is not an area where you can afford to compromise. Start hydrating today, and your body will thank you on your next hike.

Chapter 9. The Art of Meal Planning for Long Hikes

Understanding how to plan your meals for long hikes is not just about selecting tasty options to enjoy along the trail. It is a comprehensively strategic task that encompasses taking into account your body's nutritional needs, identifying lightweight yet high-quality food options, considering the food's preparation time, and ensuring you have sufficient hydration. It is an art that, once mastered, significantly bolsters your stamina and leaves you less susceptible to fatigue.

9.1. Essential Nutrients: Fueling your Body

Nutrition plays a critical role in providing the necessary fuel for your body during a rigorous hike. The primary nutrients that your body contracts for energy are carbohydrates, proteins, and fats. And while all these nutrients hold their share of importance, their consumption should be optimized based on the intensity and duration of your hike.

Carbohydrates are your body's primary fuel source and hence are paramount in your meal planning. The ideal sources of carbohydrates are whole grains such as brown rice, oats, and quinoa, fruits like bananas and blueberries, and legumes including lentils and chickpeas. Remember, one gram of carbohydrates provides four calories of energy, and these should form about 45-65% of your total daily caloric intake for optimal performance.

Protein is the building block your body uses for muscle repair and recovery. To avoid fatigue and muscle breakdown, incorporate sources of lean proteins into your meal plans, such as lean meats, fish, poultry, eggs, cheese, milk, and plant-based proteins. The recommended daily protein intake ranges from 10% to 35% of your total calories, depending on your body weight and the intensity of the hike.

Fats are a dense source of energy, providing nine calories per gram. Beneficial in long, low to moderate intensity hikes, fats should contribute to about 20-35% of your total caloric intake. Avocados, nuts, seeds, olives, and fatty fish are excellent sources of healthy fats.

9.2. Hydration: Vital for Sustained Energy

Hydration is an integral part of meal planning for hiking. It not only helps maintain your body's fluid balance but also aids digestion, nutrient absorption, and temperature regulation. For effective hydration, you should drink small amounts of water consistently throughout your hike. However, there is more to hydration than just drinking water, it also includes maintaining electrolyte balance. Electrolytes are crucial to your body's hydration process, and they influence muscle function, pH balance, and fluid regulation.

You can ensure proper electrolyte balance by including sources such as nuts (for sodium), bananas (potassium), and dairy products or fortified plant-based alternatives (for calcium). If hiking in demanding environments, consider packing some store-bought or homemade electrolyte replacement drinks.

9.3. Calculating Your Nutritional Needs

Your nutrient intake for a hiking trip should align with the hike's duration, intensity and your own fitness level. Individuals with larger body mass or higher levels of fitness require more energy than their counterparts. A rough estimate is that hiking in difficult terrain can burn anywhere from 400-550 calories per hour.

The easiest way to estimate your caloric requirement is to mildly double your non-hiking daily intake. As an example, if your normal daily calorie intake is 2000 calories, considering you hike for about 10-12 hours, your total calorie requirement would exceed 4000 calories.

Also remember that the caloric requirement will increase with the hike's altitude, temperature, load in your backpack, and individual metabolic variation.

9.4. What to Pack: Creating a Balanced Hiking Diet

When it comes to creating meals for your hiking trip, you're aiming for nutritious, convenient, lightweight, and non-perishable food items. Here are some practical suggestions for each meal of the day:

- Breakfast: Rolled oats with dried fruits and nuts, whole-grain cereals with powdered milk, and protein bars are excellent choices.

- Lunch: Dehydrated meals, nut butter on whole-grain tortillas or bread, jerky, and cheese (hard ones that are less prone to spoilage) are both, nutrient-dense and convenient.

- Dinner: Whole-grain pasta or rice teamed with dehydrated veggies and lean protein (like pouch tuna, salmon, or chicken) offer a satisfactory meal after a long day of hiking.

- Snacks: Trail mix, energy bars, dried fruit, and mixed nuts offer quick energy during your hike.

9.5. Preparing and Preserving the Food

Meal preparation is a crucial component of meal planning. If possible, prepare and dehydrate your meals at home to ensure quality and flavor. Vacuum-sealed meals stay fresh for longer periods, are lighter to carry, and easier to cook with just added boiling water.

Also, consider adequate food preservation strategies for perishable foods like cheese or cold cuts that need to stay cool as much as possible. One approach is to consume these items within the first day or two of your trip.

9.6. Trash Management

"Take only pictures, leave only footprints" should be the rule while hiking. Carry sturdy, leak-proof trash bags to collect all inorganic waste. As a responsible hiker, proper trash disposal is just as important as meal planning.

Meal planning for long hikes requires a careful juggle between nutrition, palatability, and weight considerations. But with the right planning and mix of food, it can significantly enhance your hiking experience. Like any art, it requires practice to perfect, but once you get the hang of it, the reward is immeasurable – incredible outdoor experiences fueled by delicious and nutritious meals.

Chapter 10. Recovery Nutrition: Replenishing After a Hike

After an exhilarating hike, the body needs nutrition to replenish the lost nutrients and repair the muscles that have worked so hard. Just like a car needs fuel to function, your body needs to refuel after burning off energy during a hike. Let's explore this concept with an intricate analysis.

10.1. Understanding Your Body

Physically demanding activities such as hiking stress the body, especially the muscles and immune system. It's essential to understand what happens in your body during and after a hike. Intense physical exertion uses up the glycogen stored in your muscles and liver. Glycogen is the primary fuel source during exercise, and when it's exhausted, the body fatigues, impairing performance.

After your hike, the body enters a recovery phase, replacing the lost glycogen, repairing tissue damage, and strengthening the muscles in readiness for future hikes. Importantly, the food and fluids you consume play a crucial role in this recovery process.

10.2. Essential Nutrients for Recovery

To replenish your body post-hike, you need to focus on three essential nutrients: carbohydrates, proteins, and fluids.

10.2.1. Carbohydrates

Carbohydrates are the primary food source your body uses to replenish the diminished glycogen stores. Therefore, consuming foods rich in carbohydrates soon after your hike prompts your body to store more glycogen than usual, a process known as supercompensation.

Ideally, aim to consume about 1.2g of carbohydrates per kilogram of body weight within an hour of finishing your hike, and continue to do so every 2-3 hours for up to six hours.

Examples of high-carbohydrate foods include bananas, dates, quinoa, whole-wheat bread, oatmeal and sweet potatoes.

10.2.2. Proteins

Proteins are vital for muscle recovery and strengthening. During your hike, the muscles sustain micro-tears. Proteins are essential building blocks for repairing these damages and building stronger and more robust muscle fibers in preparation for the next hike.

Aim for approximately 0.2-0.4g of protein per kilogram of body weight within 60 minutes of ending your hike.

Protein-rich foods include Greek yogurt, eggs, cheese, lean meats (such as turkey or chicken), fish, and plant-based options like lentils and chickpeas.

10.2.3. Fluids

Replacing lost fluids and electrolytes is another vital post-hike nutrition aspect. You lose a significant amount of fluids through sweating during the hike. This loss can cause dehydration, leading to fatigue, dizziness, and decreased performance.

Remember to drink water or sports drinks immediately after the hike, and keep hydrating throughout the day. The aim is to replace 125-150% of the estimated fluid loss.

10.3. Putting it together: Post-Hike Meals and Snacks

Planning your post-hike meals and snacks helps speed up the recovery process. The idea is to have a balance of proteins, carbohydrates, and fluids. Here are a few options to consider: - A smoothie made with fresh fruits (like bananas or berries), Greek yogurt, a splash of milk (or a non-dairy substitute), and a scoop of protein powder. - A whole grain wrap or sandwich with lean meat or cheese, alongside a portion of fruit. - Scrambled eggs on a slice of whole grain bread with a side of fruit.

Alternatively, if your hike ends late and it's close to dinner time, opt for a balanced full meal. Include a good source of protein (fish, chicken), a portion of carbohydrates (brown rice, quinoa), and some vegetables.

10.4. Post-Hike Nutrition for Multi-Day Hikes

For those embarking on multi-day hikes, recovery nutrition takes a slightly different turn. You must refuel at the end of each day while also preparing yourself for the next day's hike. The same principles of consuming carbohydrates, proteins, and ample fluids hold. Still, you might need to increase your intake depending on the length and intensity of the following day's hike.

So, remember to pack high-protein, high-carbohydrate, and hydrating foods suitable for preparing at your campsite.

10.5. Conclusion

Recovery nutrition is just as important as the nutrition you focus on during your hike. By replenishing your body with important nutrients — carbohydrates, proteins, and fluids — after a hike, you pave the way for faster recovery, better performance, and overall health maintenance. With the right post-hike nutrition strategy, you can continue to take on the trails, experience new adventures, and enjoy the wonders of the great outdoors.

Taking to the trails with a mindful approach towards nutrition will not only enhance your hiking experience but also contribute to a healthier, more active lifestyle. Replenish, recover, and ready yourself for the next hike!

Chapter 11. Conquering the Trails: Case Studies of Professionals

It's a brisk downwind trail in Colorado as our first expert, Harold Palmer, strategically navigates uneven rocky terrain. Once a seasoned military officer, Harold transitioned into professional hiking over a decade ago, hiking across America's most challenging terrains. He firmly believes that hydration and natural nutrition played pivotal roles in his trail-conquering stories.

11.1. Harold Palmer: The Colorado Peak Experience

Starting his ascent at 6 a.m., Harold depended on his bodily rhythm and meticulously rehearsed nutritional intake. He followed a hydration scheme, consuming 500ml of water every hour. Adding an electrolyte tablet to his water every other bottle provided the much-needed salt his body required to maintain equilibrium, crucial during vigorous physical exertion.

His food supply, predominantly plant-based snacks, included nuts, dried fruits, and energy bars. He noted avocados as his "secret weapon" for their high monounsaturated fat content, providing long-term energy release.

11.2. Lori Peterson: Adventure in the Alaskan Wilderness

Next, we turn our attention to Lori Peterson, a professional hiker known for her articulate planning and resolute determination. Lori's most recent expedition was a grueling trek through the expansive Alaskan wilderness.

Water purification methods were pivotal on her journey, as she relied heavily on collected rainwater and stream water. Using a portable water filter, she ensured that the water she consumed was free from bacteria and harmful substances.

She relied on a high-protein diet, complete with smoked salmon, jerky, and whole grain crackers. Small amounts of dark chocolate served not only as a treat but provided a useful kick of caffeine and energy.

11.3. Richard McAllister: Sierra Nevada, the Golden State's Crown Jewel

Richard McAllister, a world-renowned professional hiker, boasts of his breathtaking experience hiking through Sierra Nevada. His effective hydration habits, paired with calculated nutrition, aided his triumphant completion of the trials.

Richard sipped water throughout his hiking expedition, equating hydration with breathing - necessary and constant. He added a splash of apple cider vinegar to his morning hydration cocktail for its alkalizing properties, aiding muscular endurance.

His nourishment comprised lightweight, energy-dense foods. Freeze-dried meals were a go-to for dinner, saving on weight but delivering on the energy front. His trail mix – filled with almonds, walnuts, dried cherries, and mini dark chocolate chips – served as a powerful source of energy and a moral booster when fatigue threatened to halt his progress.

11.4. Eleanor Gonzalez: The Grande Randonnée, France

Last but not least, we meet Eleanor Gonzalez. A master of long-distance hiking, Eleanor recently accomplished the incredible Grande Randonnée in France. Her meticulous hydration and nutrition protocols sustained her energy and focus throughout the demanding endeavor.

Eleanor maintained hydration by consuming not just pure water, but also herbal teas to vary taste and gain from different herbs' benefits. Her electrolyte solution included a homemade blend of sea salt, lemon juice, and honey.

Her primary sources of energy were whole wheat tortillas, hard cheese, almonds, and dried fruits. When she needed a quick boost, honey sticks, packed with easily digestible carbohydrates, delivered a speedy energy rush.

Each of these professionals demonstrates an essential truth: the right plan for hydration and nutrition can mean the difference between thriving and merely surviving. Their stories and strategies illustrate the necessity of a well-planned regimen, expertly balancing hydration needs with proper intake of natural nutritional sources. By taking a leaf from their maps, future hikers can arm themselves with the knowledge and tools necessary to conquer their trails, turning daunting endeavors into successful journeys.